Published by medicinetraditions.com

isbn: 978-0-6488478-1-6

© medicinetraditions 2020
all rights reserved

Disclaimer

This book is not meant to treat or diagnose medical conditions. Some of the information
contained could be dangerous if used by the untrained. The author and publisher take no
responsibility for any use or misuse of the information contained.

CONTENTS

OF
BLOOD-LETTING
AND THE
Diseases to be cured thereby.

What Blood-letting or Phlebotomy is?

It is an Universal evacuation of fullness of Humours or Plethory. And Plethory is the increase of humours above equality in the Veins. The knowledge of Complexions is requisite to Phlebotomy.

The signs of a Sanguine complex are contained in these Verses:

By nature they are fat and love to hear,
News and reports, to drink and to make good cheer,
To court fair Ladies, and to laugh and sing,
And play the Poets, and learn anything,
To Wrath not prone, but noble, kind and free,
Abounding much in liberatilie,
Of red Complexion like the fragrant Rose,
And bold as Hector to affront their foes.

Signs of Plethory and Blood abounding:

When Blood abounds the face is over red,
The eyes dart out, and cheeks are fully red,
The body is unwildly, pulse is quick,
Full, soft, and in the forehead there does stick,
A tearing pain, the belly it is bound,
The tongue is dry, with thirst, and sleep profound,
Spittle is sweet, and when they sharp things take,
The taste is sweet, it cannot no difference make.

Signs of the Choleric Complexion and of Choler abounding:

Choler's humour reigns in furious men,

1

That strive to lord it over their brethren;
They learn but slowly, but can eat apace,
From whence they grow, is stature, and in face.
And heart are bold, still soaring above all,
Crafty, deceitful, angry, prodigal,
Slender, rough, dry, and yellow in their skin.
If tongue be parched with heat, and noise within,
The ears, with watching, and with vomiting,
And thirst, fat stools, and pain, and belly wring,
With loathing, heartache, want of appetite;
If pulse be hard, and swift, and hot, and light,
Mouth dry and bitter, and of fire thou dream,
Be sure the Choler is in the supreme.

Signs phlegmatic Complexion, and of Phlegm abounding:

Phlegm makes men strong; so stature broad and low,
They flatter then the Sanguine men do grow,
They idleness affect, their sense is dull,
And in much sleep they do their bodies lull,
They move as slowly as the housed snail,
And are of colour, very wane and pale,
Phlegm makes unsavoury taste, which meat does loath,
With spitting; pain in head and stomach both,
The pulse is seldom, slow, and soft, and wide,
With dreams of water, where the phlegm does guide.

Signs of Melancholic Complexion, and of Melancholy abounding:

It makes men evil, sad, and slow to speak,
To be contemplative, and sleep to break,
To be solved; but think nothing fast,
Envy and avarice in them does last.
Deceit and fear, the colour of their skin
Is sad and black, pulse hard, and urine thin.
They dream, of Ghosts, Hobgoblins and Cells,
They yawn and belch, from wind that in them dwells,
They spit and spawle, and relish very sour,
And in their left ear is a noise each hour.

What Age is fit for Phlebotomy:

Before the seventeenth year draw none at all,
In middle age oft for the Surgeons call.
Old folk, and children must but little bleed,
And then when as there is apparent need.

An addition:

At this time in great necessity, especially in a Pleurisy and other strong diseases we bleed with good success; in the fourth or fifth year three or four ounces. The middle age is from thirty to forty five or fifty.

What things hinder Phlebotomy:

Bleed not at all, when the Complexion is cold,
Nor in cold weather, nor when pain does hold
With violence, nor after thou hast been
In baths, or sporting with thy Fancy's queen,
Nor after tedious sickness, nor when
Thou art by meat or drink a shame to men.
Bleed not too young, nor when thou art too old,
Nor when thy stomachs weak with sense of cold.

Addition:

To these add: Bleed not in the beginning of a Disease, for the Crisis is the day of the motion of sickness, or in the fit, nor before the Guts are cleansed from excrements, nor in the time of the Natural courses of women, nor in the flux of the Hemorrhoids; nor after a Choleric disease, and the like, of which we shall speak in the Aphorisms for bleeding.

At what time Bleeding is good:

In every month thou lawfully may bleed,
If blood abound, and thou a vent does need,
April and May the Liver Vein is best
September's for the Spleen; and for the rest
In Winter take the Vein comes from the Head
And in Autumn let the Feet be bled
In Summer, open still the Liver vein
In Spring, that of the Heart called Median.

3

What is to be done in Bleedings

When you let Blood make a large orifice to let out the Wind and the Blood more freely, after Bleeding let him not sleep for six hours: make not too deep an orifice, least thou prick a Nerve, and let him not eat presently after Bleeding. It is good to bath two or three days afore Bleeding and three or four days after, give Wine afore and in time of Bleeding, if you fear Swooning, more before and after by gentle walking.

What is to be avoided after Bleeding

Abstain from milk, meats and drink, and cold things, and keep from foul weather: clear Air is good and rest; for motion often hurts.

Of the Effects and profit of Phlebotomy

It cheers the Sad, appeases the Angry; and keeps Lovers from madness: it clears the Sight, and makes the Brain warm, and the Marrow. It purges the Bowels, Stomach and Belly, purifies the Senses, causes Sleep. It mends the Hearing, and Voice and increases Strength.

What Vein is to be opened safely, and profit bleeding brings.

I. *The Vein between the Eyebrows in the middle of the Forehead, called* **Recta** *or* **Preparata** *is opened*

Against old infirmities, foul Ulcers, and Leprosy, Scab, Morphew, Impetigo, Itch, diseases of the Eyes, old Headache, heaviness behind in the Head, diseases of the Brain, Madness.

II. *The two twisting Veins in the Temples are opened either of them*

Against the half Headache, great Headache, and long sickness, old sore Eyes, blear Eyes, mists in the Eyes, spots, films, tears and webs in the Eyes, scabs in the Eye-lids, Nyctilops, and to make Barrenness.

III. *The Vein against the little corner of the Eye is opened a little above the jugal bone*

Against diseases of the Eyes, Head diseases abated, Headache, half Head-ache, Pannus, Tears, old sore Eyes, Nyctilops, scabs in the Eyebrows.

IV. *The Veins about or behind the Ears in the*
hollow, which appear when the Throat is tied,
and are in that place where you may feel a
beating with your finger are opened

Against half Headache, old Catarrhs, scald head, refresh and restore the memory, ulcers in the Ears and Neck, to cleanse the Face, against Toothache from defluxion, the head open, and against Ulcers and all Pain.

V. *The Vein in the tip of the Nose between*
the two gristles is opened

Against Frenzies, sharp Fevers, old Headaches, old red Faces, diseases of the Eyes and Bleareyedness, heaviness of the Head, Hemorrhoids, Itching of the Nose, Apostume of the Nose, Bother.

VI. *The two visible Veins under the Tongue*
are opened

Against Impostumations of the throat and mouth, and other Distempers there, and Quinsey after the Head vein is first opened, of impostumes in the Almonds, heaviness of Tongue, Apoplexy, Toothache, and diseases of the Gums, Catarrhs, Pannus, Cough, and distempers in the Jaws and Cheeks.

VII. *The Vein between the Skin and lower*
Lip is opened

Against stinking breath, Corrosion of the Gums and rottenness, Ulcers of the Nose, and distempers in the Face and Nose, pains in Women's breasts and Headache.

VII. *The Veins in the Lips are opened*

Against Impostumes of the Mouth and Gums, the Head vein being first opened. Against want of Breath and Leprosy.

IX. *The two Veins in the sides of the Neck,*
called Gindegi, they grow large in Singing
men, and when men hold their breath, if the
Neck be bound with a Towel are opened.

Against *Impetigo* or *Serpigo* or Itch, *Noli me Tangere* or Canker; swollen Gums, Quinsey, Asthma, Hoarseness, Impostumes of the Lungs, Dyspnoea, fits of the Spleen, side pains.

X. *The Head vein called* **Cephalica humeraria,** *and* **Cubit** *between the Thumb and fore finger without danger is opened there, and in the upper part of bending of the Arm*

Against hot pains of the Heart, half Headache, Madness, Flux of the Eyes, Epilepsy, all Diseases in the Ears, Tumour in the Head, all hurts in the Tongue and distempers of the Stomach, and Fevers if it be opened in both hands.

XI. *The Median in the middle of the bending of the Arm, between the* **Head vein** *and the* **Basilic** *or* **Liver vein;** *It is called the* **Common, Black,** *or* **Heart** *vein is opened*

Against evacuation of all Humours and hot distempers of the whole body, all Diseases in the Heart, lost Appetite, all Passions; of the Ribs, Stomach, Spleen, Liver, Sides, Lungs, Breast, and whole body.

XII. *The* **Basilic Vein** *which is called the* **Great Vein,** *or* **Inward** *or* **Liver vein** *is opened for evacuation and all Diseases*

In the Liver, Breast, Lungs, Stomach, Spleen, Pleura, against Choler from the Liver too hot, Toothache, or pain of the Back, Ribs, Sides, and all the members, Bleeding of the Nose, and Fevers.

XIII. *The* **Salvatella** *or Veins called* **Scelles** *or* **Spleen vein,** *between the ring and little finger, is opened safely in the right hand for*

Stoppage and diseases of the Liver; and in the left hand, for diseases of the Spleen: it is good also against evacuations and Diseases of the Spleen, Liver, Breast, Voice and Stomach, Heartache, Jaundice, all Fevers, stoppage of the Breast, want of Appetite, distempers in the Face, Paleness, and yellowness of the Eyes.

XIV. *The Ham vein called* **Vena Poplitis** *under the Knee in the bending is better to be opened than the Saphena*

To provoke the Terms, against pain in the Fundament and Loins, Hemorrhoids, and pain in the Bladder and Stones and Feet, all Gout or Joint pains.

XV. *The* **Sciatica vein** *in the Ankle of both Feet or thereabout is to be opened*

Against Sciatica, Gout, Elephantiasis or Leprosy, Varices, pains in the Bladder, Dysuria or difficulty of Urine, Ulcers and swellings in the Stones, and swellings, and Ulcers of the Kidneys and the like.

XVI. *The* **Saphena** *under the inward Ankle of both Feet, sometimes upon the Ankle, or on the sides of it, is often opened*

Against all passions of the Mother, and of the Stones; against old Scabs and Salt Phlegm, pains of the Hips and Legs to provokes the Terms, and Hemorr-hoids, to purge the Womb, Afterbirth, to take away Barrenness; against Diseases of the Yard and Stones, to draw blood from the Mother, Yard and Stones.

XVII. *The Vein in both Insteps upon the great Toe is opened*

Against Diseases of the Bladder, and spots in the Face, Opthalmia or sore Eyes, redness and Bleareyedness, Cancer and Varices or Veins in the Legs, and Diseases which the Saphena is opened against.

XVIII. *The Veins in both the little Toes are opened*

Against hurts in the Reins, Heaviness and Weariness of Limbs, Apoplexy, Palsy and Epilepsy.

A

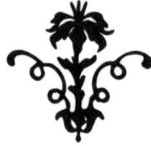

Catalogue Alphabetical
OF ALL
Diseases that may, and ought to be cured by Phlebotomy

A

1. **Abortion** to avoid it, open the Median in the first months.
2. Against *Alcola* or **Impostume in the mouth**, open the Vein in the Lips.
3. *Anchus*, open the Sciatica.
4. Against *Anhalitus* or **difficult breathing**, open the *Gindegi* or Veins on each side of the throat, or the Veins under the tongue.
5. *Anhelitus foetor* or **stinking breath**, open the Vein under the Chin.
6. Against *Angina* or **Quinsey**, first open the Head vein and then these under the tongue, or *Gindegi* in the neck.
7. **Almonds impostumated**, open the vein under the tongue above the Chin, or both Veins under the Tongue.
8. *Animi deliquium* or **Swooning**, open the Vein in the middle of the Forehead.
9. *Anus* or **Fundament**, if it be distempered, open one of the four Veins above the Groins on both sides. If pained, open the Saphena. If inflamed, open that of the Arm. If there be a hot Impostume, open the Basilic.
10. Against **Apostumes of the Anus**, if cold, open the Head vein in the Hand. If it come forth, open the Vein under the Ankle and the Salvatella.
11. Against the **Appetite dog-like**, open the *Salvatella* on the left Foot.
12. **Apoplexy**, open the Ham vein or Ankle vein, or Humeraria in the bending of the Arm, or that between the Thumb and Forefinger, or let the Nose bleed. If you first open the Saphena, and then that in the tip of the Nose it does wonders. Or open the two Cephalics, or the two veins in both little Toes, or them under the Tongue.

13. Against **Apostumes internal**, open the Median

14. **Apostumes of the Liver**, see *Jecur* or *Hepar*.

15. **Apostumes and pain of the Kidneys, Loins, Thighs, Hips, Bladder,** open the Veins under both knees.

16. **Arthritic, Articular, or Joint pains,** open first the Basilic, then the Saphena, or Sciatic vein; and the right Basilic, if it be on the right side, and the left, if on the left. If it be on the Hand, open the Sciatica on the same side, or the Ham vein.

17. Against **Asthma**, open the Median on the right side, if it be from Blood, if from Vapours on the left side; or the two veins on each side of the Neck; or open the veins under the Tongue, or the Basilic, or internal Vein in the Arm.

18. *Auditus* or **Hearing to quicken**, open the beating Vein, or that on both sides of the Nose.

19. *Aurium dolores*, or **diseases of the Ear**, open the Veins in the Temples, or first the Cephalic on the contrary side, and then on the same side.

20. If **Blood flow out of the Ears**, open the Cephalica on the contrary side. If there be an **Ulcer**, open the hearing Vein, or about the Ear. If **inflammation and Almonds**, open that under the Ear. If there be **noise** or **deafness** begun, open the vein about the Ear.

21. Against *Axillarum tumorem*, or **Swelling in the Armpits**, open the inward vein of the left Arm, if it swell not, to the bending of the Arm.

B

22. **Bilious or Choleric Humours**, are evacuated by opening the internal Vein in the Arm.

23. *Bilis atra* or **Melancholy**, by the inward Vein on the left Arm.

C

24. Against *Calculus* or **Stone in the Kidneys**, open the Sciatic vein, or Saphena in the Ankle on both feet.

25. *Calculus* or **Stone in the Bladder**, open the Saphena's.

26. *Calor* or **Natural heat abounding**, open the Vein by the Thumb.

27. In Diseases *Capita*, or **of the Head** both internal and external, open the Humerary Vein, or Cephalic in the right Arm, if on the right side, and the left, if on the left, or that between the Thumb and the Forefinger, or the Nose, or the Vein under the Chin. Or that under the Tongue; or the external Jugular *Vena Puppis*, or the Cephalica of the left Hand, or those of

the Temples, or the Salvatella; for **pain before in the Head**, open that in the middle of the Forehead; for **Fevers with Headache**, open the Median. For **old Headache**, the frontal vein or the Arteries behind the Ears, or the Temple Veins; In **Catarrhs**, open *Vena Puppis*, or those under the Tongue, or that in the Nose, or about the Ears. External Jugular, or those on both sides of the Nose, or the four Palate veins. Against **heaviness**, or **pain behind the Head**, open the Frontal vein. Against **Ulcers** and **Scabs in the Head**, open the Nose vein, or in the Temples, or about the Ears. Against **Trembling, Giddiness** and **Pain**, open the Vein in the Hollow of the Ear. Against **Melancholy**, open that between the Thumb and the Forefinger on the right hand.

28. Against **Carus**, first open the Head, then the black or Median Vein.

29. *Cephalaea* or **old Headache**, open the Forehead vein, or them behind the Ears.

30. *Cerebri passiones*, or **Diseases of the Brain**, open the Veins in the Neck or the Salvatella, or Spleen veins, Nose veins, or frontal Vein.

31. Against *Cogitations fantastic*, open the Vein in the forehead.

32. **Choleric Blood**, open the two Veins in the little Toes.

33. **Choleric heat** that between the Thumb and right forefinger, or both.

34. **Colic**, the right Basilic.

35. *Collum* or **Neck ulcerated**, the Vein about the Ear, if swollen the Thumb vein.

36. Against Diseases *Cordis* **of the Heart**; in all Passions, the Median, Salvatella and the Artery. **Trembling and Palpitation**, the internal Vein of the left Arm, the Saphena, and then the Basilic, thirdly apply Cupping glasses to the left shoulders. In **Repletion**, open the right Basilic, in **Vapours**, open the left Basilic, in **oppression of the Heart**, the Median, in **Apostume**, the Basilic or the Artery.

37. Against Diseases *Costarum* **of the Ribs**, open the Median pricking in the short Ribs the Salvatella.

38. *Coxendicum* **of the Hips**, the Saphena and Sciatica.

39. **Crudities**, the inward Veins in both Arms.

40. In Diseases *Crurum* **of the Legs, Heaviness**, the Ham or Sciatic vein. **Pain and Apostume**, the Veins in the great Toes, the Hams and Saphena. In **Swelling**, the Saphena. In **Inflammations of the legs**, the Arm veins.

D

41. In **Delirium or Doting**, open the humerary in the Arm, or the Vein between the Thumb and the Forefinger, or the Nose.

42. In Diseases *Dentium* **of the Teeth**, open the Cephalic on the Contrary side, the Palate vein, first the Shoulder veins, then under the Hips. Those behind the Ears, under the Tongue. If the **lower Teeth ache**, that under the Chin, in **pain and putrefaction**, that between the Chin and under the Lip.

43. In **Diarrhea**, open the left Basilic.

44. In **Diaphragm Inflamed and Ulcerated**, open the inward Vein on the left Arm. And in all Diseases below the Diaphragm, the Basilic, and above, the Cephalic.

45. In *Dolour* or **pain of the Kidneys, Loins, Feet, Thighs, Bladder**, open the Ham Vein; of the Back, first the Basilic then the Sciatic. If there be **Plethory**, in the joints and Feet, the Ham Vein. See *Articulorum dolour* or Joint pain.

46. In **Dysentery**, open the Liver vein on the right side if there be Repletion.

47. In **Dyspnoea**, open the *Gindegi* in the Neck.

E

48. In *Elephantiasis* or **Leprosy**, open the Salvatella on the contrary side, and then the Ham Vein or Sciatic.

49. In **Empyema**, open the Black Veins on that side.

50. In *Hepatis* or **Liver diseases**, open Basilica or Salvatella on the right Hand in a **Sanguine Impostume**, the Basilic or Cephalic, or Saphena on the same side, or the right Basilic. See *Jecur*.

51. In **Epilepsy** or Falling Sickness, open first the Saphena then the Cephalic, thirdly that under the Tongue. Also the Ham or Ankle vein, or left hand Cephalic, or left Salvatella.

52. In **Erysipelas**, open that between the Thumb and forefinger in the right hand.

F

53. In **Diseases of the Face, as Flux** and other Passions, that in the Forehead. In **Tumours, Knobs, Redness**, open the Palate vein and Cephalic on both Hands. In **Leprosy, Redness, Pustules**, that under the Chin, the Frontal. Those behind the Ears, the two Veins in the first joint of the Great Toe, the Palate Veins. In **Redness, Pustules, Spots and Ill colour**, the Frontal. In **Deformity, Foulness, Spots, Scabs, Pustules**. And either Vein in the little Toe, that behind the Ear or in the Temples, under the Chin or Tongue.

54. In **all Fevers**, the Salvatella on the left hand, or both, or both Cephalics. In **Fevers** *Synoch* the internal right Arm vein. In **Women with Child**, the Saphena and Ham in a **burning Pestilent Fever. Tertian, Quotidian, Intermitting and Semi-tertian**, the inward Vein of the right Arm. In **all Quartans**, the inward Vein in the left Arm.

55. In **Fistulas**, the Lip veins.

56. In **Fluxes, with Plethory**, the Cephalic on the right Hand, and that in the Arm first, and then that in the Ham, as Sciatica, also the Black Vein, Head Vein under the Tongue. When the **feet have water**, the Sciatica, or that under the little Toe. The **Nose**, the Saphena on the same side, and the Cephalic. In a **flux of the Belly of Blood** not excoriating, open the Black Vein or the Basilic. If it be **from the Veins of the Upper Gut**, open the Basilic or Salvatella on the same side, or the Axillaries under the Belly.

57. In *Flatus* **or Wind of the Belly**, the Cephalic.

58. In *Foetor* or **Stink and Putrefaction of the Teeth or Gums**, that in the Chin and lower Lip.

G

59. In *Genitalium morbis*, or **Diseases of the Privities**, the Sciatica, Popletica or Saphena.

60. In **Gums diseased**, first the Humerary, then under the Lips and Tongue. If **impostumated**, first the Cephalic, then the Lips. If **Pain, or Impostume, or Ulcers**, open the Veins in the Neck or Lips. In **Putrefaction, Stink, Ulcer, Inflammation**, that between the Lips and Chin, or that in the corner of both Lips.

61. In *Gibbosity*, the Basilic.

62. In **Gonorrhea**, the Basilic.

63. In Diseases *Guttaris* of the **Throat Swollen** &c. the veins of the Palate under the Tongue, the Jugulars.

64. In Passions of the *Gurgulion* or **Wheezing**, the two under the Tongue.

H

65. **Hemorrhoids, to open** them the Saphena, Ham, Sciatica or Ankle vein.

66. **Hemorrhoids to Stop**, that in the Arm called Basilic right or left, the left Salvatella is better, the Lip veins or that in the Nose.

67. In *Hemicrana* the Cephalic, Temple veins, or behind the Ears, the Frontal, the veins behind the Head.

68. *Humerorum morbis,* or **diseases of the Shoulder** that on top of the Arm, in Tumour; the left Internal, unless it reach to the Elbow.

69. In **Humours crude**: the internal vein on both Arms.

70. In *Hydrops* or **Dropsy**: the two Ham veins, or that under the Prepuce in **general swelling**: or the Cephalic **if it be wind**.

71. In **Hypochondries distempered** the Salvatella on the right Hand.

I

72. In **Jaundice Yellow**, the right Salvatella whether a Fever or no: or the Basilic; Jaundice Black, the left Basilic, and then the Salvatella.

73. In Jecoris morbis, or Diseases of the Liver; the Salvatella on the left hand, the Basilic on the right in an Impostume: see Apostume by fall or stroke, the Basilic on the other side, or the same in a Phlegmatic Impostume, the right Basilic, or on the same side in obstruction. First the black Vein, then the Basilic, and right Salvatella. If inflammation of it in the inward Vein of the right Arm.

74. In Impetigo the frontal.

75. Inflammations, first in the Arm, if that does not prevail, then in the Ham or foot: If it be a light inflammation, open the Vein beneath on the same side.

76. In Inflammations under the Reins open the inward Vein of the Arm on the same side.

77. (Inflammation) of the Fundament, Privities, Bladder, Groins, Thigh, open the upper Vein in the Arm.

78. Inflammation of the Groin the upper Vein in the Arms.

79. Insania or Madness, the Humerary vein in the Arm, the Cephalic or the Nose, Vena Puppis or in the cavity of the Ear, or in the crown of the Head, or in the Frontal.

80. Joint pain and diseases, see Arthritis.

81. Ischias or Sciatica, the Sciatic Vein.

L

82. In Lachrimae, tears or flux of the Eyes, open the Temples, the Humerary on the same side, or that Vein in the great corner of the Eye; see Oculus or Eye.

83. Lactis abundantia or Milk abounding, first the Saphena, then Scarify the Thighs and open the Basilic.

84. Lassitude or Laziness of Limbs, the Ham Veins.

85. Laterum dolour or side pain, the Gindegi or Median.

86. Lentigo, the tip of the Nose, or that in the Lips, or under the Chin.

87. Leprosy, the frontal or Gindegi in the Neck.

88. To lighten the body and mind, the Vein of the Prepuce.

89. To lighten the feet and legs, the Ham vein.

90. In diseases Linguae of the Tongue, in Impostumes, Tumours, first the Cephalic on the right side, then the Lip veins or under the Tongue. In slowness or hindrance of speech, the vein under the Tongue, or when it is swollen the veins under it, or the Cephalic.

91. Lipothymia or Swooning, the Frontal.

92. Lippitude or Bleareyedness and redness &c. open the veins between the Thumb and forefinger, or the Cephalic of the left hand, or the tip of the Nose, or in the Temples, or in the corners of the Eyes.

93. Loins pained and other Diseases, both the Hams, the Median, the Saphena, both the great Toe veins, and the Sciatica.

M

94. In Mammillarum or Pap diseases, open the Vein under the Chin. When the Paps are swollen or impostumated, the Saphena.

95. Madness; first the Basilic, then the Median or Saphena, the Cephalic, or Humerary in the Arm, in the Nose; see Insania or Madness.

96. In Mother diseases, open the Salvatella in the left hand, the Sciatica or Saphena. When there is an Ulcer or Impostume, open first the Basilic, then the Saphena. When there are Clefts, the left Basilic or left Saphena. When a Cancer, first the Basilic, then the Saphena. In an Inflammation, open the Ham or Ankle vein. When there is Itch, open first the Median, then the Basilic. When it is discolored upwards, open the Saphena. When Fallen down, the Basilic. When it is Suffocated, the Saphena or Ham vein: to purge and cleanse the Mother, open the Saphena.

97. Maxillarum affectibus or in diseases of the Jaws, first open the Humerary veins, then under the Lip and the Veins of the Palate.

98. In the Diseases of the under Jaw and Mandible, open that under the Tongue: when they are swollen, open the Gindegi and the veins above the Ears.

99. Melancholy, open the right Cephalic or the left Vein of the Back, the left Basilic, or first the black Vein, then the Basilic or Foot Vein.

100. Memory to repair and keep it open, the veins behind the Ears, or the Nose vein.

101. Menstrua or Terms to provoke, the Saphena and that behind the Clavicula or the Knee vein, or that in the Ham: or first open the Basilic, then both the Saphenas, or open one one day and the other the next, and take four ounces: or open the vein in the Great toe, or that in the little Toe, or the Sciatic vein.

102. To stop (the Terms) open the Basilic.

103. Mictus sanguinis or Pissing of Blood, open the Basilic and Saphena, or the Cephalic, if it bleed from the Bladder, Liver or Spleen: if bleeding come from the Reins, Kidneys, or back, open the Saphena.

104. Mole, open the Saphena often.

105. Morphew, open the Frontal, or vein in the Nose, or that under the Chin.

N

106. Nostrils bleeding, open the Saphena on the same side, then the Cephalic, in Bother or Itch open the Nose vein in an Ulcer the Saphena; if the Terms or Hemorrhoids begin to flow, if not open the Cephalic and Nose vein, or that under the Chin: if they stick open, the Cephalic and then the Nose vein.

107. Nerves when weak, the Ham vein.

108. Nyctilops, the Cephalic or lachrymal veins in the Nose, then in the Temples, or the Arteries behind the Ears.

O

109. Occiput or the hinder part of the Head pained, open the Vein under the Tongue, the Vena Puppis, or of the neck.

110. Oculi the Eyes, in their Diseases, open the upper Vein in the Arm, those in the Temples, that in the Forehead, or under the Thumb, or first the Cephalic, then the Frontal, or in the corners of the Eyes. In pain or dim sight, open the great Toe vein, or them in the corners of the Eyes by the Nose: in spots of the Eyes and redness, the Nose vein; in Lippitude, Catarrhs, Clouds, Dimness, Moisture, &c. open the Temple veins on both sides, the right Cephalic, both Veins in the great corners of the Eyes. In heaviness, open the Frontal, in Redness, the Nose, in heat and pricking, those in the corners of the Eyes.

111. In Tears, Defluxions and Moisture, the Humerary on the same side, or that in the great corner of the Eye, both Cephalics, both the Temple veins, and that of the Nose.

112. In Lippitude, that between the thumb and the forefinger in both hands, the Nose vein, and both Temples, both the Veins, and in the great corners of the Eyes near the Nose, the left Cephalic: in Tumour or Ulcer, both the veins between the Thumb and the forefinger, both the great Toe veins, and that in the middle of the Forehead: in inflammation and salt Tears, open the Humerary on the same side, or that in the great corner of the Eye.

113. Omnes humores or all humours, to purge and cure all Diseases. If the blood offend, open the Median.

114. In all Diseases of the Nutritive members, open the Sciatica or Saphena.

115. In all Diseases above the Diaphragm, open the Cephalic.

116. In all Diseases in parts under the Diaphragm, the Basilic.

117. Opthalmia, the Cephalic in the contrary hand; if there be Plethory, first the opposite Basilic, then the Cephalic, or first the Saphena on the same side if the matter be little and a Flux, the Cephalic on the same side, also the Temple veins, or them in the great Toe, or between the Thumb and forefinger, or Arteries behind the Ears.

118. Orifice of the Stomach pained, the Artery is to be opened.

119. Oris or Mouth evils, the Tongue veins, in pain, the Palate vein; Stink, that under the Chin, or that between the Chin and Lip, or that in the hollow of the Ears: in Impostumes and Ulcers, first the Cephalic, then the Lip veins, and under the Tongue.

P

120. Palpebrae or Eyebrow if Scabby, the Cephalic or Lachrymal veins, or of the Temples, if thick, the Cephalic.

121. Palpitation of the Heart: the inward veins of the left Arm.

122. Pannus the Temple veins, and the two Arteries behind the Ears.

123. Palsy: both the veins in the little Toes, or that under the Tongue.

124. Parotis: that under the Ear.

125. Pectoris of the Breast: the Basilic on the left Arm, the Neck veins, or the two under the Tongue.

126. To cleanse the Breast: open the Salvatella.

127. Pedum or Feet, in all pains open the Ham vein, or in the little Toes, when swollen and red, the Ham and Sciatic veins. In Itch and Scabs, the two great Toe veins.

128. Peripneumonia: the Basilic opposite; if the pain reach to the Throat, Breast or Arm, open the Internal Vein on the same side.

129. Percussion or Stroke causing impostume: the Basilic

130. Pestilent Fever: the right Arms inward vein.

131. Plague, if it be in the Neck: open behind the Ears; if in the Cervix, the Cephalic in the Arm or Thumb. If in the Chin or Forehead, the veins under the Tongue.

  If in the Head, Shoulder, Breast, the Median.

  If in the Arms, Ribs, Breasts, Armpits, the Basilic, Median & Salvatella.

  If in the Thigh, the Saphena.

  If in the Knees, Shins or Ankles, the Sciatic vein.

  If in the Loins and Feet: open the Palsy vein near the little Toe.

132. Phrenzie, first the Hand Cephalic, or the Saphena which is better, then the Forehead: but take heed that he move not much in, or after bleeding, or the humerary, or between the Thumb and Forefinger, or in the Nose.

133. Phthisis or Consumption, first the left Basilic, then the Salvatella.

134. Pleurisy, the opposite Basilic, at the beginning when the matter flows, when there is plenitude; or first open the Saphena, and then the Basilic. If it be in the right side, open the right Saphena, when there is but little plenitude, or when the matter is flowed, then open on the same side, or the Gindegi and Median. If the pain reach to the Throat, Paps or Arm, open the internal Vein on the same side.

135. Plethory, when no part is affected any Vein may be opened with benefit. In Plethory that makes diseases from unknown causes, open the Liver vein in the right Arm. Plethory of crude humours, in internal Veins in both Arms. Plethory from Terms stopped, the Saphena. Plethory great with Defluxion, first the Veins in the Arm; and if that will not do, the Leg or Foot veins. Plethory of Melancholy, the inward Vein in the left Arm. Plethory of Choler, the inward Vein in the right Arm.

136. Podagra or Foot Gout, first the Basilic, then the Arthritic or Saphena: and the right Basilic, if it be in the right Foot, if in the left, the left; also the Ham vein. See Arthritis.

137. Podex inflamed, the upper Veins in the Arm.

138. Pregnantes, or Women with Child, bleed about the fifteenth week, again when they open again about the twenty sixth week, open the Hepatic against the little Finger. Andrenatus allows to Plethoric women with child, bleeding in the second, third or fourth month, but not in the eighth or ninth month.

139. Priapism, first the black Vein, then the Basilic.

140. Pudendi or Privities, the Saphena, the Genital vein, Sciatica, Ham vein, or the Veins above the Pecten. When there is Ulcer or Tumour, open the great Toe veins. See Virga.

141. Puerpura or Women with Child in Fevers, open Saphena and Ham veins.

142. Pulmonum or Diseases of the Lungs, the Median; the Veins under the Tongue, the inward Vein in the left Arm, the Salvatella. In impostumes of the Lungs, the Gindegi.

143. Punction or pricking under the small Ribs, the Salvatella.

144. Pupil of the Eye dilated, the Cephalic or Lachrymal Veins, and the Temples.

Q

145. Quartan Ague, the inward Vein in the left Arm.

146. Quotidian daily, Intermitting, and the Seminary, the inward Vein of the right Arm.

R

147. Rhagades or Clefts of the Womb, open the Basilic in the left Hand, or the Saphena in the left Foot.

148. Raucedo or Hoarseness, the Gindegi, the two Veins on both sides the Throat near the Neck.

149. Reins, in all Diseases, the left Salvatella, the Veins in the Knees, the Vein in the Glans of the Yard. In pain present or to come, the right Basilic, then both Saphenas. In plenitude, the Ham vein or Ankle. In obstruction, the Basilic often, then the Saphena. To evacuate and mundify, the Sciatic, to strengthen the Veins between the Loins and Buttocks. In inflammation, the inward Vein of the right Arm, if the right Kidney, suffer in the left, if the left Scabs, the Basilic. Apostumes and Ulcers, the common vein if there be Repletion: or the Basilic on the same side, if the humours offend, or the Cephalic, if the matter be above. Or the Saphena on the same side, and the Ham vein. In the Stone, the four veins above above the Pecten, or the Sciatica.

150. Rheum: the Palate vein.

151. Rheum upon the Eyes sharp: the Temporal Arteries must be opened.

S

152. Sanguinis in Blood abounding and unclean: open the Basilic or right Salvatella, or the little Toe when it is hot and choleric: open both little Toe

veins. When there is Melancholy: open the Veins between the Loins and Buttocks.

153. Scab or Itch: open both little Toe veins.

154. Sciatica: the Sciatic vein on the same side, Saphena or Ham vein.

155. Speech hindered: the veins under the Tongue.

156. Sleep profound, first the Cephalic, then the Median.

157. Spatula or Shoulder diseases: open the vein in the top of the Arm.

158. Spiration with difficulty and the like: that under the Tongue, the Median and Salvatella.

159. In Spleen diseases: open the inward Vein in the left Arm, Gindegi: first the left Basilic, then the Salvatella, or the Sciatica and Saphena.

160. Spondil Diseases: the Vein in the top of the Arm.

161. Spitting of Blood: the Saphena, with Ulcers, the inward vein on the left Arm.

162. Spitting of Blood from Terms stopped: open the Basilic twice or thrice, or the Saphena once.

163. Spitting of Matter: the Black vein on the same side.

164. In Sterility or Barrenness from moisture: both Saphenas.

165. Stomach Passions: the Median, Basilic, and the vein of the under Lip.

166. Stomach Impostumes: the right hand Basilic, if Plethory be first the Saphena, then the Basilic or Median.

167. Stomach Evil complexion with matter: the black vein, if there be Plethory.

168. Stomach Orifice hurt, the Salvatella.

169. Stupor: first the Basilic, then the Cephalic, then that vein that is proper to the numbed member.

170. Subet from Blood: first the Cephalic, then the Black vein.

171. Synanche or Quinsey: first the Humecaries under the Tongue, or both Cephalics, then the Gindegi.

172. Syncope or Swooning: the vein in the forehead.

173. Synoch Fever Simple and Putrid: the inward vein of the right Arm.

T

174. In Tabes or Consumption: the Inward left vein: see Phthisis.

175. Tenesmus: the right Basilic, or the left, if there be Repletion of Blood.

176. Tertian Burning, Pestilent, Quotidian, Constant or Intermitting, and Semi-tertian: open the Inward vein in the right Arm.

177. Testicles or the Stones, to empty the Saphena. In diseases of them, both the veins on the sides of the Pecten, or that in the knee. In pain, the

Saphena. Tumour or inflation, both Saphenas, the Sciatica, the Groin vein, both great Toe veins. In impostumes of the Stones, the right hand veins, if pain or impostume be on the right side, after that the Saphena on the same side; if the impostume be on both sides, in both sides. In a wound of the Testicles: the Basilic, especially if there be Repletion.

178. Thorax or Breast: open the internal Cephalic of the left Arm. See Pectus or Breast.

179. Tibiae or Legs pained: the Ham or sciatic vein.

180. Trembling of Heart: the Saphena then the Basilic, thirdly apply Cupping glasses to the left shoulder. In Repletion, open the right Basilic, in vapours the left.

181. In Tristitia or Sadness: the Cephalic.

182. Tumours of all sorts: the Groin vein and Cephalic.

183. Tumours in the Armpits or shoulders: the inward vein of the left Arm.

184. Tumours of Tongue and Jaws: the right Cephalic.

185. Tussis or Cough: the Cephalic, if matter fall; or the Black vein, if there be matter contained; or the Basilic, if the Liver being hot cause it; or the Saphena, if the Terms be stopped.

186. If blood be coughed up: open the inward vein on the left Arm.

V

187. In Varices: open the Sciatica, Saphena or Ham vein.

188. Venter or Belly diseases: the Basilic. In Belly flux: see Diarrhea or Fluxes.

189. In Vertigo or Migraine: the Cephalic, Ham or Ankle vein, or the Arteries behind the Ears.

190. Vesica or Bladder offended: open the veins on each side the privities or Saphena. If it be impostumed: the left Basilic or left Salvatella. If inflamed: the upper veins in the Arm. If a Stone in the Bladder: see Calculus.

191. In Virgae or the Yard diseases: the Sciatica, Saphena, Ham the four Veins above the Pecten, the Basilic on the same side. In inflammation, open the upper veins in the Arm. Tumour or Ulcer, both the great Toe veins.

192. Visus or sight weakened from many Spirits: first open the Basilic, then the Cephalic; if there be great Repletion, take first the Saphena. If it be from the Spleen, open the left Cephalic. See Oculus.

193. Vomica or impostumes: open the two veins in the little Toes.

194. Vomiting: the Head, or black vein, or Basilic, when there is Choler. If blood abound, open the left Basilic or the Saphena; if the Liver cause it, open the right side Basilic.

195. Voice hurt: the Salvatella or veins under the Tongue.

196. Urine difficult, the Basilic and then the Saphena, or the veins on both sides the privities. See Mictus or Pissing.

197. In Uteri malis or diseases of the Womb, open the Salvatella of the left Hand, Sciatica or Saphena. In inflammation of it, open the Ham or Ankle vein.

198. Uvula fallen: open the right Cephalic or Basilic, if there be Repletion.

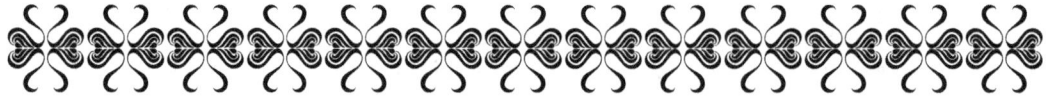

APHORISMS

TO BE

Observed in Bloodletting

Hippocrates his Aphorisms
concerning Phlebotomy

1. If the Vessels be emptied as they should be, it does good; and the patient likes it well, if otherwise not. Therefore consider the Climate, Time and Age, and Diseases, whether you ought to bleed or no.

2. All diseases by Repletion, are cured by Evacuation or Blood-letting, if large and violent, or much at the nose.

3. If any be dumb on the sudden, open the vein in the right arm.

4. A woman with child will miscarry upon bleeding, and the sooner as her child is older.

5. In acute diseases open a vein, when the disease is vehement, and the patient in his youth and strong.

6. The veins behind the Ears being opened, cause Barrenness.

7. If you will let blood, by reason there is blood gathered together, to turn it from the place, do it at a great distance from the part afflicted.

8. The opening of the veins beneath in the Groins, Thighs, Legs and Ankles, makes men unfruitful.

9. It is good for a man to bleed sometimes: the time of bleeding begins at February, and again at September.

The Aphorisms of *Galen*

concerning Bleeding

1. There are three considerations in Blood-letting; the vehemency of the Disease; the youth of the Patient; and the strength of the Faculty.

2. Nor too young, nor too old are to be let Blood.

3. They need no Blood-letting that have natural evacuation.

4. Many need bleeding after long Diseases by the three considerations mentioned

5. We Bleed when there is no fullness, when there is great pain, or in a Fracture or dislocation; or any contraction in a Joint.

6. Bleeding requires strength agreeable to the Evacuation.

7. It is not good to Bleed often in a year.

8. When you let blood, keep off far from the Artery.

9. Bleeding and Water-drinking are chief remedies of continuing Fevers.

10. When you will cure obstructions first open a Vein though there be no fullness.

11. Necessity allows and commands Blood-letting at any time or hour.

12. It is a good Remedy in continual Fevers to let Blood till they faint, if the Patient be strong.

13. Two hours after Bleeding the Patient may eat.

14. In Bleeding in continual Fevers consider not the number of Days, but only the strength.

15. If at the time of bleeding the Terms chance to flow, or the Hemorrhoids, observe it, and if the quantity voided be sufficient, leave the whole business to Nature and that flux, but otherwise bleed a little.

16. These are inconveniences that follow: loss of blood, Faintness, worse habit of body, a colder temper, discolouring of the whole body, and falling into long deadly diseases.

17. In all Fevers bleed at the first if the patient be strong.

18. It is lawful by bleeding to evacuate superfluities in a Fever.

19. In a Phlegmon of the Liver, the blood that flows thicker must be let out by opening the internal Vein in the right arm.

20. In a Frenzy and Lethargy, bleed at first coming of it.

21. In a Carbuncle bleed till they faint.

22. In great diseases, always bleed, but with respect to the age and the strength.

23. You must bleed plentifully in a Lassitude with a Phlegmon, sometimes till they faint.

24. After bleeding you must not presently refresh the Patient.

25. Abstain from bleeding when the blood is good and little, and other humours are abundant; but when it is contrary let blood.

26. If you forbear bleeding by reason of the age or for fear, let the Patient purge the more.

27. To open the Hemorrhoids, or provoke Terms, open the Ankle vein, and then purge is good with bleeding in the Arm.

28. When blood abounds, it must not presently be let out: for fasting, slender diet, looseness of belly, or purging, or bathing often, or exercise alone, or much rubbing will abate it.

29. After the opportunity of bleeding is passed, other evacuations are dangerous when there are excrements either in the Brain or the Instruments of the Spirits.

30. Bleeding must be at the beginning of Diseases, and sometimes purging.

31. Bleeding is a common way to cure diseases by Repletion.

32. Bleeding whatsoever, or wheresoever, or howsoever done, equally evacuates the whole body.

The Aphorisms of Cornelius
Celsus *out of his* Book 2.
Chap. 9.

1. There is scarce a Disease in which bleeding is not allowed.

2. It is an old custom to let blood in young men and women not with child.

3. But not Children and old folks, and Women with Child; for the Ancients thought the first and last age could not endure this kind of help, and were persuaded that if Women with Child should be let blood, she would abort; but after this, Custom has showed that it is otherwise; for it is not material what age the party is of, or what is in the body, but what strength the Patient is of.

4. Therefore, if a Youth be weak, or if the Women be not with Child, and be also weak; it is not good to let blood, for so the strength that remains will be taken away: but a strong Boy or old Man, and a hearty strong Woman with Child may be cured by bleeding according to Celsus.

5. But the Physician may be deceived if unskilful, because in those ages there is less strength.

6. A Woman with Child has need of strength after her cure, not only for herself, but to sustain the Child.

7. The chief art is to consider the strength of a Child, old Man, or Woman with Child.

8. There is difference to be observed between a fat and a lean body, a strong and a weak.

9. The thin bodies have more blood, the full bodies have more flesh.

10. They endure the loss of blood better, and a fat man is sooner disturbed with it if it be too much.

11. Therefore the strength of the body is better to be found by the Veins than the form.

12. Nor are these only to be considered; but the Disease; what kind it is, whether abundance or want of matter hurts; whether the body be corrupt or sound.

13. For if the matter be wanting, or be sound, that is another thing: but if it offend in plenty or be corrupt, it can no way be better helped than by bleeding.

14. Therefore in a vehement Fever when the body is red, and the Veins are swollen, bleeding is required.

15. But if the Fever be vehement, and you let blood in the height of it, you kill the patient.

16. Therefore, expect a remission: if it decreases not, but has ceased to decrease and you hope for no remission, then though it be worse bleeding then before, avoid not the opportunity.

17. Sometimes make two days work of it, if there be necessity, for it is better first to refresh the Patient, and then do it thoroughly, then to spend all the strength at once.

18. If you bleed for the whole body, open the Arm; if for a part, bleed in that part, or near it. But this cannot be done everywhere, but in the Temples, Arms, or about the Ankles.

19. Some say that blood must be drawn far off from the part affected. For that will divert the course of the matter, and take away that which offends. But that is false; for it empties the nearest part first, and blood flows thither from the remote while it bleeds: when it is stopped it will not be drawn. And experience shows, that if the head be broken, that it is best to bleed in the Arm.

20. If there be fault in the shoulder, the contrary Arm is to be bled, because if there be any evil, the part that is affected will sooner receive it. Sometimes blood is diverted when it breaks out in one part, and you let blood in another. And it ceases to flow by applying things that stop to the part, first bleeding, and giving it another vent.

21. Though bleeding be easy to an Artist, yet it is hard to an ignorant person. For the vein is joined to the arteries and the Nerves to them. Therefore, if the Lancet touch the Nerve, there is stretching of the Nerve, which is grievous.

22. But an Artery cut, neither grows together, nor will be healed, but sometimes causes a violent flux; but if a Vein be cut, the heads or orifices being pressed down the blood stops.

23. If the Lancet be fearfully applied, it only cuts the Skin, not the Vein.

24. The Vein must be cut in the middle out of which when blood flows you must observe the colour and habit of body; for if blood be thick and black, it is bad and fit to be lost. If it be red and shining, it is sound, and the loss of it (instead of profit) hurts; therefore it must be stopped.

25. But these things cannot happen to a Physician that knows what Body ought to loose Blood.

26. If it be all black, let it often out, and bleed not again, if you have enough before fainting.

27. Tie up the arm with a Pledget dipped in cold water, and open the vein with your nail the next day, for the new Escar will easily come off, and it will bleed again.

28. But whether it be in the first or second day, that blood which first was thick and black, begins to wax red and clear, there is enough taken; therefore let the Vein be presently bound up, and kept so till there be a strong Escar which will quickly be in a Vein.

The *APHORISMS* OF
Arnoldus de Villa nova
out of his Book of the Regiment of Health.

1. After Bathing, or Venery, or great Exercise, bleed not by any means.

2. And also after long sickness.

3. They which serve in hot houses, and take great pains in their calling to resolve the Body, must not be let blood.

4. Bleed not in very hot nor very cold Weather.

5. The Spring and Autumn are best times to let blood in.

6. Bleed not in Pestilent Air, cloudy, or stormy Weather, or when the South-wind blows.

7. In Summer bleed at eight in the morning; in Winter at noon.

8. Let young men bleed in the first Quarter of the Moon, and old in the last.

9. Sanguine men must bleed in the first Quarter; Choleric in the second; Phlegmatic in the third; and Melancholic in the fourth.

10. If the Moon be in a sign with Evil aspect, or to any member, bleed not in that member.

11. In Aries, bleed the Head; in Gemini, the Arms; in Cancer, the Median; in Sagittarius, the Thigh; in Aquarius, the Legs and Thighs; and in Pisces, the Feet. The other parts are safe at any time.

12. If the Moon be in Taurus, Virgo, Capricorn, it is bad to let blood; if in Cancer, Scorpio, Pisces, indifferent; if in Aries, Libra, Sagittarius or Aquarius it is good.

13. Let Drunkards and Gluttons, and those that are filled to loathing, abstain from Bleeding.

14. If any want Blood-letting, and neglect it there will be Impostumes, inward and outward, the great and small Scab, the Ringworm, Synochus, Measles, Apoplexy and Palsy, Small Pox and Spitting of Blood, Quinsey, Plague, sudden Death and Leprosy, and generally all sickness of much blood or corruption of Blood; and they that are inclinable to such Diseases, let them not neglect Phlebotomy.

15. There are many Evils by bleeding unreasonably. From often bleeding come Obstructions, Dropsies, Age hastens on, the Appetite decays, and

Stomach, weakness of Heart and Liver, Trembling and Palsy, and weakness of all virtues both Natural and Animal.

16. He that is very musculous and fleshy, by accident, and he that is extenuated, and they which use to diet that breeds much blood, and live in idleness and pleasure, and dwell in Countries where there is little resolution, and that eat much flesh roasted, and drink sweet Wines, and use Baths, and no copulation, and exercise little, are more to bleed than others, and they who fast and eat Melancholic meats are to bleed less.

17. When Phlebotomy is used to evacuate and in a place near the Diseases of the part where it is, then the first blood ought to be worse than the second, and the second then the third; and if the contrary happen, there is still need of bleeding and Physic. But in some bodies that need little bleeding, it often happens that the first is better than the second, and then you may bleed again presently.

18. Before bleeding it is good to exercise, move and watch to make it move better. The Member to bleed is to be rubbed and heated, and washed with warm Water, to make the Vein plainer and the blood freer.

19. The Surgeon must be young, expert, and of quick sight, not trembling or drunk.

20. If a weak hearted patient, or one very faint is to bleed, let him first eat Bread and drink astringent Wine.

21. They whose blood is thick, immovable, and the Veins hidden, must be bathed for some days before, except the body be very plethoric.

22. Before bleeding let the Belly and Bladder be free.

23. In those that have an Impostume bleed while the colour of it changes: but when there is a simple plenitude without an Impostume, except not the change of blood, for the blood may be all alike, or good.

24. If the Blood be whitish and thin, lose but little.

25. In Summer and Spring bleed in the right side; in Autumn and Winter in the left.

26. In a venomous matter, bleed on the same side.

27. When there is great necessity open the same Vein twice in a day, or when you have not taken enough.

28. If after the Vein is opened the Blood will not flow, then it is good to cough and hawk, and clap the patient upon the Shoulders.

29. Touch the Blood as it comes forth, if it be cold, stop it presently, and also if it be very hot and thin, for in both cases, you may fear Swooning.

30. Take a drop of blood upon the Nail, if it flow off, and stand not firm, it is waterish, and must be presently stopped.

31. Or drop it into water; if it sink, it is too thick, and if it disperse and swim, it is too watery; if it be in a mean, it is good.

32. After bleeding, Exercise not that day but rejoice at home, nor Bath that day, and use no Venery till the fourth day, not sleep in the day.

33. Consider also the substance of the Blood; it is either Melancholic, Phlegmatic, Sanguine, Pure, Choleric, or Watery.

34. Melancholy is the dregs of blood, it is black, and in the bottom of the Poringer; and when there is too much of this, it is no good sign, then we may judge that the Patient is sad, envious, and curious, fearful and poor-spirited; such must use things to cleanse and increase Blood.

35. Phlegm is white, slimy, unsavoury, like whites of Eggs, and it is in the blood next above the Melancholy; this must not be too much, and if there be much of it, we judge him to be Phlegmatic naturally, sleepy, rude, and dull to action, and to spit much; but there ought to be more of this than of Melancholy.

36. Then follows pure blood; it ought to be of a purple colour, reddish or ruddy, of this there ought to be more; if there be much of it the Patient is Sanguine, and free, amiable and cheerful, laughing and of a red colour, bold and bountiful.

37. Then follows Choler which is the froth of Blood; of a Saffron colour, with glittering red; there ought to be less of this than of Blood or Phlegm, and more than of Melancholy. If there there be great quantity of this, we may judge the party Choleric, and by consequence crafty, deceitful, wrathful, bold and prodigal, apt for action, watchful and subtle.

38. Moreover you must consider the watery substance that swims at top when the blood is congealed, as whey when milk is curdled, and it is like Urine, if it be put into a Glass; and when this water is like the urine of a sound man whose blood it is, it is good; otherwise not.

39. And when this water is separated more perfectly from the blood, the better it is, and the better is the digestion and decoction in the Liver. And the contrary.

40. This water must be in the blood to make it thin, that it may pass more free through the great Veins and small, and to come to the members. Therefore it is not good that blood should be without this water.

41. For it wanted show, dryness and thickness of blood, this is in such as fast much, and watch, and eat dry and hot meats, and that study and exercise much, and in some that are well.

42. Moreover it is not good that too much water be in the blood, for it would show defect of digestion, either in respect of meat or drink, or in respect of the parts that cannot convert the meat into blood, and it shows also too much coldness and moistness of blood, and weakness of body.

43. Hence it is that they who have cold Stomachs, and Livers, and Veins, and eat cold and moist Meats, and much, and especially drink much, and exercise little, and fast not, nor watch, have such blood.

44. Also in blood there is a fleshy substance declining to white, for the Blood beginning to whiten in the Veins, because the farther digestion to convert it into Members proceeds in whitening. This digestion begins in the great veins, and end in the small with the Members of the third Digestion, namely at the outward solid members of the whole body.

45. This substance is flesh-like, and appears manifestly in Blood after it is washed, and the fatter, moister, or more watery the Blood is, the less there is in it of this substance, and the thicker (except it exceed the temper) and less fat, and without water, the more of this fleshy substance is to be seen.

46. Therefore from a great quantity of this white substance, is signified the good digestion in the Veins, and the pliableness of the Blood to turn into Members, especially when you feel it with your hands. And when there are no great things contained in it, that are not hard, but will crumble with the fingers. For by such there is signified an inclination to a Leprosy.

47. Moreover if thou would know the substance of the whole blood, cut it when it is congealed with a knife or thin stick, and if it resist not but cut easily, it signifies the subtlety of the Blood; but if it divide with difficulty, then it signifies sliminess and grossness of Blood.

48. And if Blood will not cut, though it be easily divided as it is in Oil, and water and other moist things which are easily divided, though not cut, that blood is too thin, and that thinness argues want of digestion.

49. And when blood is easily pricked but not cut then it is slimy, and that Blood is commonly Phlegmatic.

50. And when it is cut but with resistance, then the blood is gross, but not viscous or clammy.

51. You must consider also of the colour of blood; for if in one part of the Poringer it appears one colour, and in another of another colour, as in a Pigeons neck, it signifies diversities of Evil humours.

52. Therefore we must consider the true fixed colour of the blood; it is red and purple, not dark red, and that argues good Blood.

53. If it be a glittering red, it argues predominant Choler, and also if it be like Saffron. If it be frothy, it shows wind. If it be white or livid, or blue, it signifies cold predominant Phlegm, and especially if the blood be slimy, and there are other signs of Phlegm.

54. These colours may come from burning, as appears in Consumptive and Leprous persons. Green signifies burning, and especially Choler; Black and Blue signifies natural Melancholy, or that which is burnt.

55. You may also consider the taste, for it ought to be sweet; if it be unsavoury, it signifies Phlegm predominant; if bitter, Choler; if sour or brackish, Melancholy and sour Phlegm; if it be salt, it signifies salt Phlegm and adustion of Humours.

56. The scent is also to be considered; if it be sweet and pleasant, it is good; if it stink, it shows great putrefaction in the humours.

57. Moreover if blood be drawn do quickly coagulate or congeal, it is too gross; if it be long and slow to congeal, it is too thin and undigested.

58. If it be in a mean, the blood is indifferent.

APHORISMS of *Avicen,*
Rhasis, Aetius, Montagnanus,
Savanarola and *Damascen,*
and others.

1. They that use much Blood-letting in Youth, are cured after sixty sooner than others, and their natural heat is choked, especially if they are of a cold complexion.

2. They who dwell in the fourth or sixth climate, may lose more blood than they that live in the Seventh, First, second or third.

3. They who have weak Stomachs, and cold weak Hearts and Livers, and Cold, and have cold Diseases, must not let blood; nor Melancholic persons, except their Veins be swollen. Nor pale, lean, starved, or such as eat Melancholic food, nor such as use too much Venery, nor such as have a Dysentery or Iliac, or are much bound in Belly, nor such as have not bodies prepared, nor such as are seventy, except they be strong, and have broad full veins, and used it, and when there is necessity.

4. At sixty open not the Cephalic.

5. At fifty open not the Median.

6. At seventy take heed of opening the black Vein.

7. It is good for Phlegmatic persons to open a Vein when the Moon is in Aries or Sagittarius.

8. For Melancholic, when she is in Libra or Aquarius.

9. For Choleric, when she is in Cancer or Pisces.

10. In the New and Full, abstain from Phlebotomy.

11. Let youths from fourteen to twenty-five bleed in the first Quarter.

12. From twenty-five to thirty-five, in the second.

13. Bleed in the morning when the Sun is risen after an hour, two, or more of sleep.

14. After noon, open the Head, Hand, and Feet veins, and the Arms in the morning.

15. Let old and sick people eat Broth and drink wine an hour or two before.

16. They who sweat easily and often want Blood-letting.

17. Usual accustomed Bleeding is not to be omitted without danger.

18. After Bleeding, drink thin and good Wine: avoid Mead, Ale, Fish, and what breeds bad blood.

19. Bleeding when there is no necessity does more harm than good.

20. After Bleeding, avoid bad Air, eat white Bread, well baked Veal, Hens, Chickens, lamb, roar Eggs, and that which breeds good humours and blood, drink pure Wine clear and thin; abstain from Cheese, Milk, Herbs, Fish, Ale, and Mirth, Anger, Sadness and Copulation.

FINIS

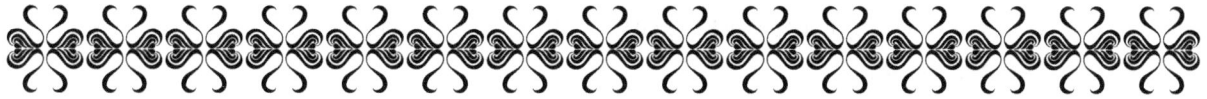

OF
CUPPING
AND
SCARIFYING,
And Diseases cured thereby

The Time and Age of Cupping
and Scarifying

1. Scarify not before four years old, nor after sixty.
2. Cup not nor Scarify in the Full or New Moon.
3. It is good when the Moon is in Cancer, Libra, Scorpio, Aquarius and Pisces: but not in other signs. It is good in the second or third hour of the day, and after an hour they may eat and drink.
4. Let the body or part to be scarified, be washed an hour, or half an hour with hot water before and rubbed.
5. It is good to use Cupping glasses after Evacuation of the Body. For it is not good in Plethory, or to any part that has a Flegmon.

The Use and Profit of Cupping
in General

Cupping without Scarification

1. Is good to turn an Impostume from a noble part to an ignoble or inferior part.
2. To draw heat to a Member weakened by Cold.

3. Against the Colic, if applied below or above the Navel.

4. To take away Pain.

5. Against Dislocations.

6. To draw out that which lies deep to the skin outward.

7. To evacuate Wind and Humours.

8. To stop the Flux and Hemorrhoids.

9. To heat a Member, and to draw Blood and Heat to it.

10. To reduce a Member into its place.

11. Against pain of the Matrix, if they be fastened under the Navel and the Woman sit warm with them upon her.

12. Against extraordinary Flux of the Terms, if applied under both Breasts an hour or more.

13. Against Bleeding at the nose, applied to the Liver, if the right Nostril bleed, and upon the Spleen, if the left.

14. Against a Pestilent Botch to draw venom from within.

15. Against a Rupture in the Groin.

16. To divert Blood that flows immoderately from any part or place.

17. To stop the fluxes of the Stomach.

18. To stop Blood, applied to the opposite parts.

19. To attract Blood, extract Poison.

20. Against a Cold Stomach, if applied to it.

21. To remove Wind.

The Use of Cupping-glasses with
or without Scarification, according to Places and Parts

Cupping-glasses upon the Head;
are good

Against Madness, Dizziness, Baldness, Scabs in the Eyes, Bother, sticking out of the nape of the Neck, and other Diseases. But

They hurt

The Understanding, Memory. Cause astonishment, and hasten Madness in dry Brains.

Cupping-glasses to the Forehead,
are good

Against pain in the hinder-part of the Head, heaviness of Head and Swelling, diseases of the Brain, Madness and Doting.

They are good to the Forehead,
for the Face
In old diseases of it, Impetigo, Ulcers, Leprosy, Scabs, Morphew; And also diseases of the Eyes and Migraine. But,
They hurt
The Reason and Understanding.

Under the Chin, they are good
Against Pustules and Tumours in the Mouth, Tooth diseases and Gums; Spots in the Face, and the like. Against the infirmities in the skin; of the Head, Throat, Jaws, Cheeks.

Applied to the Back-bone between
the Neck and Shoulders
Against diseases in the Head, Face, Neck, Teeth, Nostrils, Eyes and Mouth; Heaviness, Impetigo, Quinsey, and are instead of opening the Cephalic or Median. But,
They hurt
The Memory, and make the head shake.

Applied between the Shoulders, right against
the Heart and Stomach, they are good
Against diseases of the Breast, Neck, Shoulders; against Asthmas, Cramp, Trembling of Heart from blood, and diseases in the Throat, and are instead of opening the Basilic. But,
They hurt
The Stomach and Heart, and make a trembling without blood.

Under the Breast, they are good
Against diseases thereof, and Asthma.

Upon the Liver
If it be dry or inflamed.

Upon the Back
Against Diseases there.

Upon the Stomach, they are good
Against Tumour in it, cold and foul Humours.

Upon the Hands
Against all diseases of the Head, Eyes and Ears.

Upon the Kidneys and Reins
Against Impostumes of the Hips and Scabs, and Hemorrhoids, Gout, Leprosy, Itch and Scabs of the Back; Wind in the Mother, and other cold Wind in the Bladder, diseases of the Thighs, and all parts beneath.

Under the Navel
Against diseases of the Matrix, Colic, and Griping.

To the Hypochondria
To stop Bleeding at the Nose, and Womb.

To the Loins
They provoke the Hemorrhoid, take pain from the Back, Mother and Loins, Scabs from the Thighs, Impostumes and Tumours, and allay Venery or Lust

Upon the Buttocks
They cleanse the Blood of the whole body, and are good for the sides, Loins, and Breast, and abate Lust.

Before the Hips
They are good against Impostumes in the Stones, and starting forth of the Ribs and Hips.

To the Hinder part of the Head
They are good against Impostumes, strains in the Buttocks.

Under the Ham
Against beating in the Ham from hot humours, against Strains and Ulcers in the Legs and Feet.

To the Thighs

They are good for the whole body, against swollen and impostumed Buttocks, pains in the Kidneys, and Bladder, Fluxes of the Eyes, Diseases in the Head. Against hot burning Impostumes in the Knees, Evils in the Breast and Back. Impostumes in the Cods, applied inward to the Groin. Against wounds in the Hip, and Thighs. Against old pain in the Mother, and to purge it from Superfluities. Against Impostumes in the Hands and Strains, applied behind. To provoke Hemorrhoids and the Terms, they cleanse the Blood and take away Plethory, and are as good as any Blood-letting.

To the Soles of the Feet

They provoke the Terms, are good against the Sciatica, Gout, Migraine, and instead of Phlebotomy in the Feet veins.

A CATALOGUE

of the Diseases to be cured by Scarification and Cupping

A

1. Against **Anctae** apply them between both
2. **Angina or Quinsey**, apply them often to the shoulders with Scarification, and cup the Thighs.
3. **Anus or Arse-hole hot Impostumes**, Cup the Loins and the Upper part of the Buttocks.
4. **Anus or Fundament out**: cup the Muscles of the Back.
5. **Apoplexy**: Cup and Scarify the Neck and Shoulders, and the Thighs.
6. **Apostems and strains in the Buttocks**, Cup the Hips behind.
7. **Asthma**: Scarify between the Shoulders where the neck and the Back join together.
8. **Aurium or Ear diseases**: Cup in the Wrists and under the hinder part of the Head on both sides the Neck.
9. For **Ears bleeding**: Cup upon the Shoulders.

B

10. **Basilic vein** is as good as opened when Cupping-glasses are applied between the Shoulders under the Neck, where it is joined to the Back.

11. **Bother**: Cupping behind in the Head or Pole, or behind in the Head about the Crown, or above the Forehead is good against it.

C

12. **Canicies or Baldness**: Cup behind in the Head, and in the Crown before, or above the Forehead.

13. **Cephalic vein** is as good as opened, if you apply Cupping-glasses upon the top of the Head behind, near the Veins on the sides of the Neck that ascend to the Head.

14. **Capitis or Head-diseases**, are cured by Cupping the Neck and Shoulders with Scarification, and by Cupping upon the top of the hinder part of the Head near the two Veins in the side of the Neck that ascend to the Head, or by Cupping with Scarification in the Wrists.

15. **The Head is cleansed** by Cupping under the Chin.

16. And **upon the Fundament**, Cupping draws from the Head.

17. **Trembling of the Head**: by Cupping upon the top of the hinder part of the Head, near the two Veins in the side of the Neck that ascend to the Head.

18. **For pain in the Head behind**, Scarify the Forehead.

19. **Colic or Heart trembling**, scarify between the Shoulders.

20. **Corpus or body is refreshed**, by Cupping the Fundament.

21. **Coxae or Hips** are cured of Impostumes, Scabs and Strains, by Cupping within side, or on the Loins, or that part that contains five Spondils.

22. **For the two internal parts of the Hips**, Cup between the two Anchae.

23. **Crurum or Thighs**, are cured of Scabs, Ulcers and Strains by Cupping before in the Hips, and Scarifying under both knees.

D

24. **Delirium** to cure, Scarify the Neck and Shoulders.

25. *Dentium doloribus*, **or Toothache**, Cup under the Chin, and upon the top of the hinder part of the Head, near the two Veins on the sides of the Neck that ascend to the Head.

26. **Diarrhea**: to cure, Cup upon the Region of the Spleen.

27. **Dyspnoea or difficult breathing**, cup the Shoulders.

28. **Dolour [pain] to allay**, Cup upon the part.

29. *Dorsi dolores* **or Back pains,** upon the Loins and Back.

30. **Dolour of the Shoulders:** Cup upon the part between the Shoulder blades under the Neck, where the Neck is joined to the Back.

31. **Dolour of the Throat:** Cup in the same place upon the Throat.

32. **Dolour of the Colic;** Cup upon the Navel.

E

33. **Against Elephantiasis:** Cup the Loins or in the part that contains five Spondils. Also Scarify the Thighs and Feet.

34. **Epilepsy:** first Cup the Thighs, and then the part where the Neck is joined to the Cranium, or Cup the Shoulder blades.

F

35. **Against Face-evils:** Cup under the Chin, and upon the top of the hinder part of the Head near the two Veins in the side of the Neck that ascend to the Head.

36. **Fevers are certainly cured** by Scarifying upon the Back bone with ten or twelve Cupping-glasses.

37. **Flux and blood that corrodes** beneath: Cup with Scarification upon the Buttocks at the bottom of the Loins: or use Cupping without Scarification upon the same parts, and about the Navel, and about the right and left Hypochondria.

G

38. **Gum-evils,** Scarify under the Chin.

39. **Gibbosity,** Cup the Buttocks or the Brawn of the thighs.

40. **Gullet or Evil pain:** Cup between the Shoulder-blades under the Neck where it is joined to the back.

41. **Guttur or Throat:** Cup under the Chin.

H

42. **Hemorrhoids to move:** Cup the Loins.

43. **Hemorrhoids to stop:** Cup between the Shoulders without Scarification or with, or about the Loins and Reins which is better.

44. *Humerorum dolores* **or the Shoulder-pain**: Cup between the Shoulder-blades under the Neck where it is joined to the Back.

I

45. **Jaundice Yellow**, Cup upon the Liver, under the right Shoulder, or under the Ribs.

46. *Jecoris* **or Liver diseases**, Scarify in the Region of the Liver.

47. **Liver inflamed** and the like, Scarify the right Hypochondrium.

48. **Iliac Passion**: cup the upper part of the Belly.

49. *Insanium* **or Madness**: Scarify Neck and Shoulders, and before in the Head, about the Crown, and above the Forehead.

50. **Incontinence**: Scarify Buttocks and Loins.

51. **Intestines Evil**: Cup the Fundament.

52. *Ossis exitum* **or Bone out of Joint**: Cup upon the Anchae.

L

53. **Against** *Lactis abundantia*, **too much milk**, Scarify the Thighs.

54. **Lust**, Scarify the Loins and Back.

55. *Linguae Magnitudinem* **or Tongue too big**: Cup and Scarify upon the Shoulders in the Neck.

56. **Tongue Impostume**: Scarify behind the Ears, or Cup under the Chin and Neck.

57. *Lippitudo* **or Bleareyedness**: Scarify Neck and Shoulders.

58. **Loins disease**: Scarify the upper part of the Buttocks and the bottom of the Loins.

M

59. **Mandibles to mundify**, Cup under the Chin.

60. **Against Madness**: Scarify the Neck and Shoulders, or Cup above the Fore-head.

61. **Mother diseases**: Scarify the Thighs below, and Cup the Navel and against the Mother Windy: Cup the Loins or that part that contains five Spondils immediately among the Twelve.

62. **Mother fallen and suffocated**: Cup the Groins, Hips and Pecten.

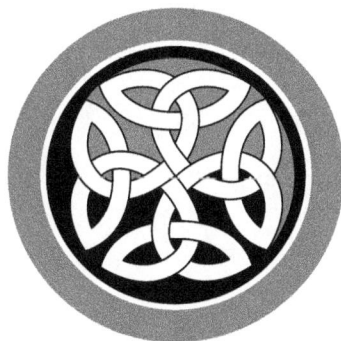

medicinetraditions.com

The ultimate resource for the
Study of Traditional Medicine

www.ingramcontent.com/pod-product-compliance
Lightning Source LLC
Chambersburg PA
CBHW080900030426

42334CB00021B/2617